7 Minu

Series
Acid Reflux
How I Cured Myself

Mae Segeti

Copyright

Copyright © 2015 Mae Segeti

Published by Skinny Stuff LLC

Disclaimer

The information included in this book is for informational and educational purposes only, and is not intended as a substitute for the medical advice of a licensed physician. I am not a medical doctor. Any advice I give is my own opinion based on my own experience. You should always seek the advice of your own health care professional before acting upon anything I recommend, publish or imply. By reading this book, you agree that my company, my partners and I are not responsible for your health or the health of your dependents or loved ones. Use of the advice and any other information contained in this book is at the sole discretion and risk of the reader.

Any statements or claims about the health benefits conferred by any foods, supplements or exercise methods have not been evaluated by the Food and Drug Administration and are therefore not intended to diagnose, treat, cure or prevent any disease.

Table of Contents

Author's Note   5
Introduction   7
ONE - How It Started   8
TWO - Suspension of Disbelief   15
THREE - What Is Acid Reflux?   18
FOUR - Possible Causes of Heartburn   20
FIVE - Benefits of Yoga   24
SIX - Letting Go 32
SEVEN - Pranayama & Asana   35
EIGHT - Meditation   48
Conclusion   49
About the Author 50
A Message from the Author   51
Bibliography   52

Author's Note

Thank you so much for purchasing my book, Acid Reflux – How I Cured Myself, the first book in the 7-Minute Solutions Series. This publication was put together with your health in mind.

I have met many people suffering from the same condition as me—acid reflux. After I discovered a solution that finally relieved my condition, I felt the need to pass this information on to anyone I thought it could benefit.

I have told people I know what I have found to be helpful, but it never seemed that I was getting through to them. At the same time, I know how incredibly common this problem is, and that most people are not lucky enough to find the same answers I have found.

In this book, I will share with you my experiences and lessons learned about coping with and managing my lifelong acid reflux. I truly hope that the information in this book helps ease your suffering.

All I ask is that you keep an open mind and give my solution a shot before passing judgment. The air you breathe is free, so practicing what I describe to you in this book is not going to cost you anything. You have nothing to lose except for the pain of acid reflux.

Please do not consider any of the following information as medical advice. Always consult your doctor before making any changes to health practices.

If this book helps you in any way, please take the time to review it.

Once again, thank you for your purchase. I wish you the best of health!

Mae Segeti

Introduction

I am not a doctor, therapist or yoga instructor; I am a sufferer of heartburn (also known as acid reflux). I have done a lot of reading and researching on the subject purely out of necessity, and have found a natural solution that I hope will work for you.

The reason acid reflux is called heartburn in English (not in most other languages) is because, sometimes, when it gets bad, you don't even feel the burning sensation—only a pressure in the chest. It can sometimes feel as if somebody very heavy is sitting on your chest. Some people say it can also be mistaken for a heart attack, but to me this pain in my chest feels more like what I imagine having an asthma attack might be like.

Through this book, I will share with you the benefits of yoga and yogic breathing, and offer clarification on the many styles of yoga out there. I will also share some of the competing theories about and causes of heartburn. I will show you the exercises that I still do every day, which seem to have kept me free of pain for many years.

ONE - How It Started

Here is my story, as it relates to acid reflux. I still remember the first time I felt it—an uneasy burning sensation running from the base of my stomach to the bottom of my throat. I did not know what it was. At first, I thought I was just hungry. It is easy to confuse heartburn with hunger: In both cases, you feel a burning discomfort in your stomach area.

I was around 11 the first time I felt it. My mom had made one of my favorite meals, a simple vegetable stew with some onions. I finished my first plate, but somehow I felt hungrier than before I started eating. I ate more, but the feeling only increased. My mom told me that what I was feeling might be heartburn; she had felt it a lot when she was expecting me. Heartburn is very common among pregnant women.

I tried all of my mom's home remedies: baking soda, popcorn and a few others I cannot recall, none of which worked for me. As time went on, I kept getting worse. Eventually, I had to start cutting foods out of my diet. First to go was soda (which was probably not a bad idea), but I even had to cut out healthy foods like apples, garlic and onions. Even seemingly harmless foods like radishes, carrots, broccoli and cauliflower had to be eaten with bread, or else my heartburn would be unbearable.

Despite the dietary changes I made, there was no improvement. By the time I was 14, doctors suspected I had an ulcer and ordered a urea breath test for Helicobacter Pylori, the bacteria that is responsible for ulcers. It required me to drink a mixture, wait some time and then exhale into a piece of equipment to see if the bacteria was growing unchecked in my body. The treatment is simple—a cycle of antibiotics—but my test came back negative. I was given many pills, such as calcium carbonate, ranitidine HCl and famotidine, along with information on what not to eat, but none of it helped.

Looking back, I realize that I had been under a lot of stress. I know that sounds silly, given that I was only 14 at the time. But I was in a special dance program at school, and there was a lot of pressure on me to give exceptional performances. I was also dealing with the constant competition common among young ballerinas, not to mention the usual pressures of adolescence.

The heartburn would not go away; it just kept getting worse. I eventually had an EGD (esophagogastroduodenoscopy) performed. In this procedure, a camera attached to a flexible tube goes down the throat to check the lining of the esophagus, stomach and the first part of the small intestine. The test itself is not painful, but it is definitely unpleasant. I did not mind. I trusted that it would finally tell me what was wrong, because by this point I could only sleep sitting up. I propped myself up every night with a bunch of pillows, which hurt my back but did not really make a difference as far as my acid reflux went. The EGD found nothing, but I was offered more pills: esomeprazole and omeprazole.

I was eating roughly 400-500 kcal/day, losing a lot of weight, and had no energy. I could only eat a few bites, and every bite caused more pain. I was taking a lot of over-the-counter medications, but they only helped for the first two weeks after starting a new brand. As soon as I got used to whatever medication I was taking at the time, the pain would start to come back.

I was accepted into a drug trial, which had already been on the market but needed further testing. It belonged to the PPI (proton pump inhibitor) group, a type of medication that shuts down some of the cells in your stomach that produce acid. The assumption is that you have too much stomach acid, and that is what might be causing your heartburn. It is logical, but it did not help me one bit.

After the first few days of taking the PPI medication, I got a little better. But around day five (I had to keep a strict diary) I started experiencing more pain than ever before, so I discontinued the medication. As soon as I stopped taking the pills, the pain started to subside. When I shared this information with the people conducting the study, they pronounced me "cured". Their reasoning was that if, at some point during the study, I could say that I felt better than I did before the study, it meant that the medication had worked. It did not seem to matter that the medication had made my discomfort and pain worse in the end.

Here I have to say that I do not mean to bad-mouth the medical profession at all. I do take pills when I get a toothache or have an infection, and I would definitely go to a hospital if I were in a car accident. However, I feel that when it comes to chronic issues such cancer, high blood pressure, arthritis, digestive issues and such, natural alternatives need to be explored. I have deep personal faith in diet, acupuncture and yoga as a possible cure.

I am in no way trying to discourage you from following your doctor's advice. All I'm trying to say is that, no matter who's giving you suggestions or directions, it is good to always use common sense instead of following blindly.

Doctors and scientists have been wrong many times in the past. Just think back to when they used to practice bloodletting, saying that too much blood in the body was the cause of poor health. Another example is Hungarian doctor Ignaz Semmelweis, who discovered the cause of puerperal fever (also known as childbed fever), a vicious infection that killed many mothers shortly after giving birth. The cause: the bacteria from the doctors' hands and tools were transferring to the women. The solution: Doctors should disinfect their hands and tools. This was a new idea in Vienna in the mid-1800s. Dr. Semmelweis lost his job and rejected by the medical community, while the unsanitary practices went on for decades.

As these examples demonstrate, contemporary science is always changing. Practices doctors used to swear by seem ridiculous today.

After years of struggle, I found the solution that changed my life. Fate—and a lot of research—eventually brought me to a wonderful old yoga teacher who taught me how to fix myself. I had to make changes in my thinking and learn to do a few exercises every day, but my stomach problems went away. I truly felt cured this time. I could even handle drinking coffee if I wanted to.

I continued to study the lessons taught by my yoga teacher and others. I quickly committed myself to learning more and more about yoga, buying copies of every yoga book I could get my hands on and signing up for as many classes as I was able to squeeze into my schedule.

Over time, I developed a short sequence of exercises. These exercises have nearly eliminated my heartburn and made an incredible change in my day-to-day life. I can now eat anything I want, although I still try to eat small dinners, as this helps me get a more restful sleep. If I do have a heavy meal of mostly cooked foods at any point in the day, I will take some digestive enzymes along with it. The only catch seems to be that if I forget to do the exercises for even just a few days, the pain gradually starts coming back.

The solution I found can best be described as learning to let go, and practicing a few specific yoga exercises (mostly breathing exercises, also known as pranayama). Do not worry, you will not have to seek out a guru in India or convert to a new religion. Anyone can do these simple exercises—anywhere —in just a few minutes. I still do these exact exercises every morning.

The only thing you need is an open mind. Western society has conditioned us to accept pharmaceuticals and surgery as the only methods of healing. These usually have unexpected and sometimes unpleasant side effects. Medications and surgery can be expensive, and are not always covered by insurance. It is also common for both medications and surgery to fail to help the patient at all.

I have had countless conversations with people over the years—including doctors—which proved to me that it is indeed hard for most people to accept any method of healing other than pills or surgery. I was once one of these people, constantly popping pills to ease my heartburn. For the most part, none of the pills gave me much relief.

Unfortunately, my wonderful old teacher has passed away. In this book, I will sum up what I have learned from her as it relates to acid reflux and heartburn.

TWO - Suspension of Disbelief

Many people around the world have set ideas about yoga. I have met several people from various religious backgrounds that do not want to have anything to do with yoga, as they see it as a pagan spiritual practice. To these people, I say, "Try to open your mind, and suspend disbelief."

Think of the last time you went to see a movie. There was probably at least one glaring plot hole that you didn't even notice because you granted the director the benefit of the doubt. You chose to go along with the experience presented to you. If you want to enjoy a movie, it is best not to obsess over the details. Rather, you should accept the world the story reveals to you. That is what I am asking you to do with this book—suspend your own beliefs and ideas. Let your mind be open to new thoughts and concepts, at least long enough to absorb what is in this book.

If you are reading this book, it is most likely because you too have suffered from heartburn, acid reflux or GERD longer than you would like, and are in search of something—anything—that can offer you relief. If nothing seems to have helped you or if you are seeking an alternative to the sometimes harmful effects of prescription medications or surgeries, then it might be worth listening to what I have to say and giving this practice an honest shot.

Yoga comes from ancient Sanskrit texts originating with the Indus-Sarasvati civilization. Hinduism and Buddhism came from the translations of these texts, but they offer much more than that. You do not have to leave your religion and convert to Hinduism to benefit from this book. You can just take a few beneficial aspects of yoga and apply them directly to your own life.

In July of 2013, the California Superior Court ruled that schools in Encinitas, CA, could use yoga classes for fitness, not to indoctrinate elementary school students into Buddhism. Judge John Meyer ruled that the practice, which originated in India, is now a "distinctly American cultural phenomenon."

The only addition I would make to this is that the United States is not the only country outside of India where yoga's popularity has grown extensively in the last few decades. Yoga has now become a worldwide tradition—it is all over Europe, Canada and some parts of the Middle East. Worldwide, people are becoming open-minded enough to enjoy the wonderful benefits of this ancient practice.

Even people living in countries largely dominated by strict religious traditions and rules have found ways of incorporating yoga into their daily lives. Did you know that yoga is very popular in Iran? In a country ruled by Sharia Law and an Islamic political system, they have the National Iranian

Yoga Association. If the Iranian people can be open-minded enough to accept the benefits of this tradition, even with perceived conflicting religious values, so should those of us in the West.

If you look at all of the major religions of the world, they pretty much strive to do the same thing: They explain where we came from and where we are going (or not going) after this life is over. With the two grand questions in life answered, our minds are open enough for our various religions to teach us a few basic guidelines for living our lives as well. That is it. All the other stuff is just getting lost in the details.

So I say that if you are so desperate to get rid of pain that you picked up this book, it is worth trying what is inside of it. Please do not let any preconceived notions of what yoga is or is not prevent you from learning something that may change your life. This is a short book, and you can do the exercises described in under 10 minutes. Do them for a few weeks and see how you feel. Try to think of this as simply a new daily exercise, like going for a walk or stretching, because that is exactly what it is.

THREE - What Is Acid Reflux?

Heartburn is a symptom, and acid reflux is the cause. You can have acid reflux without having heartburn, but there is no heartburn without acid reflux. Acid reflux occurs when, for various reasons, our bodies' natural defenses fail to protect us from our own stomach acid, allowing gastric juices to contact, burn and damage sensitive tissue. This can be incredibly painful for many people. Some people have regularly occurring acid reflux that causes them no pain at all. However, if you feel heartburn, that is the result of acid reflux. Chronic acid reflux is gastroesophageal reflux disease (GERD).

The stomach is a highly acidic environment. In our bellies, we carry a large sac of strong acid sloshing around, waiting to digest anything that comes its way. The stomach's job is essentially that of a sacrificial pit that tries to dissolve anything tossed into it, and then distribute its nutrients (and poisons) throughout the body, via the bloodstream.

The only thing keeping the stomach acid from burning holes through the stomach lining is a protective layer of mucus known as gastric mucosa, which nature saw fit to provide us with. However, this mucus lining can be compromised, and is not always able to protect us from high amounts of acid.

The key to most cases of acid reflux lies in a small muscle known as the lower esophageal sphincter (LES). This muscle is what separates the stomach from the esophagus. The esophagus lacks a protective lining of mucus, and should not have contact with the powerful acid in the stomach. The food and digestive juices leak out of the stomach and into the esophagus because the LES barrier is compromised or weakened for various reasons, resulting in acid reflux and heartburn.

FOUR - Possible Causes of Heartburn

For some people, simply cutting coffee from their diet might be all they need to do to resolve a case of heartburn. For others, it might be figuring out the source of a constant headache, relieving them of their continuous aspirin regimen. For those who have already tried everything they could think of, I offer a few more possible explanations as to why your heartburn has been plaguing you.

There are two opposing schools of thought when it comes to treating heartburn.

Conventional Medicine: Too Much Acid

This is why most doctors will give you pills and possibly other remedies to help reduce the acid in your stomach. Anyone who has struggled with heartburn long enough is familiar with at least a few of these. There are three major types of medications used to treat heartburn and acid reflux: antacids, H2 blockers and proton pump inhibitors (PPI).

Commonly known brand names for these are the following:

Antacid: Tums, Rolaids, Mylanta
H2 blockers: Tagamet, Pepcid
PPI: Nexium, Prilosec, Prevacid

I have tried various forms of all three types of medications and none of them gave me lasting relief. Instead, many actually made my condition worse, which is why I have chosen to share with you a different theory about the cause of acid reflux, as well as many other digestive issues.

Holistic Medicine: Not Enough Acid

The reasoning is that insufficient stomach acid can lead to improper digestion, resulting in the stomach becoming so full of undigested food, gas and bacteria that it pushes against the esophageal sphincter muscle, forcing it to open and release the stomach contents into the esophagus. The stomach has a lining that protects it from acid; however, the acid, along with undigested food, is not supposed to get up into the esophagus. The esophagus does not have a protective lining, allowing us to feel the pain of acid reflux. The burning in the chest is from the damage to the esophagus by the contents of the stomach. If you want to learn more about the theory behind insufficient stomach acid, try Craig Fear's wonderful book 30-Day Heartburn Solution.

If you believe the theory of not enough acid, or you are just desperate for relief, it might be beneficial for you to try a touch of lemon juice in water, or a little apple cider vinegar by itself or diluted with water. You can also take digestive enzymes or betaine HCl (hydrochloric acid) in pill form.

One thing both of these theories seem to agree on is that the stress of our modern lives and diets is one of the main causes of acid reflux.

Overeating/Pregnancy

Some people overeat on a regular basis. Having the stomach too full can cause the esophageal sphincter to open up and release the stomach contents into the esophagus.

More than half of pregnant women suffer from heartburn. A likely reason for this is the fetus taking up a lot of space and pushing on the stomach, forcing it upward.
Similarly, overweight people can have their excess fat deposits push the stomach upward, causing the same problem.

Unhealthy/Denatured Food

Currently, many people rely on already cooked foods, take-out and fast foods. Everyone is busy trying to make ends meet, so time for cooking an actual meal is limited.

When I speak of healthy eating, I refer to eating a balanced meal that does not contain ingredients that will make your heartburn worse. Processed and canned foods can be lifesavers in an emergency, but you should not eat them regularly. Cooked or denatured foods lack natural enzymes, as heating anything to 108°F (42°C) or over is going to destroy these enzymes, making it a lot harder for us to digest them.

Exercising or Sleeping on a Full Stomach

Another possible cause for heartburn can be physical activity too soon after a meal. If you try going for a jog after eating a big meal, it is possible that the muscle is not going to hold tight enough, and you might wind up suffering from heartburn.

Similarly, try not to go to bed shortly after eating. If you must, lie on your left side to prevent food and acid moving up the esophagus.

Known Irritants

Several medications, such as Aspirin and Ibuprofen (known as NSAIDs), can irritate the stomach. A simple way to avoid this is by taking them with food. In most cases, there is a warning on the label under the directions that tells you not to take it on an empty stomach. Be very careful when taking HCl in pill form on days when you also take NSAID medications—the combination of the two can possibly make heartburn worse.

FIVE - Benefits of Yoga

When some people think of yoga, they think of people twisting themselves into pretzels, and practicing difficult and often uncomfortable postures. Many of the postures seem forced and unnatural to the human body, and have no appeal to most Westerners. At first glance, yoga may seem to be solely about flexibility training. This could not be farther from the truth. Yoga is more than just flexibility. Yoga is about cleansing the body with exercise to allow the mind to become calm and reveal the True Self.

The many poses (asanas) and breath work (pranayama) of yoga were developed not only to give yogis healthy bodies, but also to train their bodies to tolerate both the physical and energetic strains of long meditation practices. The point was to train the body to care for itself while the yogi focused on important things such as advancing the mind and spirit.

If a yogi trained his body well enough, he could withstand sitting meditation practices lasting a few days. The average Westerner would probably find it difficult to meditate alongside a trained yogi. It is difficult to sit and meditate for hours if you experience physical pain and discomfort after only a few minutes. While most of us might not have the desire to spend the rest of our lives meditating, yoga still has tremendous benefits for the average person.

Anybody can practice yoga, as all poses and breathing techniques have modifications for beginners and injuries. But what I want to focus on here is the benefits it can have on your health.

There are extensive studies on the effects yoga has on health and the body. Most of these were done in India, but there are more and more studies done every year in the US and Europe—and there will only be more, as yoga's popularity continues to grow in the West.

Dr. Timothy McCall, MD, a board-certified physician and medical editor of Yoga Journal, lists 75 health conditions that benefit from yoga practice. These include:

- Alcoholism and other drug abuse
- Anxiety
- Asthma
- AD/HD
- Autism
- Back pain
- Balance problems
- Carpal tunnel syndrome
- Chronic fatigue syndrome
- Depression
- Diabetes
- Drug withdrawal
- Eating disorders
- Epilepsy
- Fatigue
- Fibromyalgia

- High blood pressure
- HIV/AIDS
- Hypothyroidism
- Inguinal hernia
- Insomnia
- Irritable bowel syndrome
- Menopausal symptoms
- Menstrual disorders
- Metabolic syndrome
- Migraine and tension headaches
- Neck pain
- Neuroses
- Obesity/overweight
- Obsessive compulsive disorder
- Osteoporosis
- Osteoarthritis
- Performance anxiety
- Post-joint replacement
- Post-traumatic stress disorder
- Psoriasis
- Restless leg syndrome
- Rheumatoid arthritis
- Rhinitis
- Schizophrenia
- Scoliosis
- Sexual function
- Sinusitis
- Smoking cessation
- Stroke
- Total knee arthroplasty
- Traumatic brain injury
- Tuberculosis
- Urinary bladder dysfunction

- Urinary stress incontinence

According to the hatha yoga tradition, positive and negative energies govern our health, and in order to have perfect health these energies need balancing. Yoga can help you find the connection between your body and mind. The body reacts to even the smallest changes in the mind. Using this connection, yoga can make your body healthy again, and the easiest way is through our breathing. Breathing exercises help to balance these energies.

Yoga says that the body does not get sick as long as it lives according to nature's ancient laws. Health is living in harmony with nature; sickness is a result of leading an unnatural life. Unfortunately, our modern society does not resemble our old ways. We do not eat, drink, breath or sleep naturally anymore. We have not done so for a long time.

Yoga can teach you to live by the rules of nature (as much as is possible in Western society).

Among many other things, yoga can improve muscle strength and flexibility, and boost mood and circulation. A lot of the asanas (yoga poses) involve what are called bandha, which is a contraction of specific muscles in the body. These contractions squeeze the blood out of a specific area, and their release sends new blood full of nutrients flooding into the area, washing out cellular waste products. This act of contraction is what is largely responsible for yoga's benefits to individual organs and improving digestion, which in our case aids in alleviating heartburn and GERD.

Different Schools/Origins of Yoga

There are many different schools of yoga, and several of them are newer, Western twists on an old tradition. None of them are right or wrong, and they all come from the same ancient roots. Many of the differences stem from people interpreting the ancient texts in different ways. By no means is what follows an all-inclusive list of the various types of yoga, but it may help guide you in choosing the right class.

Hatha Yoga

Hatha yoga is the trunk of the family tree that most yoga styles taught in the West originate from. The common Western image of yoga is technically hatha yoga. Hatha yoga (movement of the body) is one of the eight limbs of yoga described by Patanjali. Hatha yoga focuses on the practice of asanas (yoga poses). If you decide to attend a hatha yoga class in your local gym, you can generally expect a basic introduction to the exercises. The gym can be a great place for beginners. However, I have attended a handful of classes that were not labeled as advanced, yet would have been hard to follow for someone with no experience. You are in the hands of your teacher, so if you find one you like, it can be beneficial to stick with them.

Anusara Yoga

Anusara is one of the newest styles of yoga. John Friend, a teacher of Iyengar Yoga before developing his own approach, founded it in 1997.
Anusara Yoga can be a great style for a beginner, as teachers of this style honor the unique abilities of each student.

TriYoga

This little known type of yoga is a complete system based in the ancient practice. Founded by Kali Ray, a yoga master originally from the United States, it concentrates its practice on combining postures, breathing and building focus, with special emphasis placed on flowing movement.

TriYoga can be practiced at night instead of in the morning to help calm the mind, release stress and allow the body to heal itself.

Iyengar Yoga

Named after its founder B.K.S. Iyengar, who started teaching in 1936 at the age of 18, many consider this a purist style of yoga. Iyengar Yoga is a restorative method of yoga, which involves holding poses longer than in most other styles, paying great attention to proper body alignment, and frequently using props such as yoga blocks, straps, blankets, pillows and even chairs. This might be a good style for someone with health concerns, as teachers go through a rigorous training program before certification.

Ashtanga or Astanga Yoga

K. Pattabhi Jois developed Ashtanga in 1948. Ashtanga follows a set sequence of exercises that have been used for almost 70 years and been proven effective in building flexibility, strength and stamina. A great benefit of Ashtanga lies in its students being able to memorize the sequence, allowing them to flow in a manner similar to a moving meditation. Ashtanga is not recommended for beginners.

Power Yoga

Power yoga developed in the late 1980s and stems from Ashtanga. The main difference is that there is no set sequence, allowing teachers to create a unique class every time. I do not recommend this style for beginners.

Bikram

Bikram Yoga was the developed by the Indian-born Bikram Choudry, and is similar to Ashtanga yoga in terms of intensity and involving a set sequence of poses. Thus, it is not for beginners, but rather people who have advanced in their yoga practice. The main characteristic of this style is practicing in a heated room. The room is set at 105°F and 40% humidity. Bikram Yoga's 26 poses include two breathing exercises, and are done in a 90-minute session. The intense heat helps prevent injuries and detoxify the body, but people with heart conditions, high blood pressure and other health issues should avoid this style. Please make sure you consult your doctor before taking a Bikram class.

Hot Yoga

Hot Yoga is not the same as Bikram yoga, though people commonly confuse the two. Hot yoga rooms are heated, but do not require a certain temperature. They can be anywhere between 80–100 degrees, and can vary in humidity levels. There is no set sequence of poses either, allowing the teacher more freedom. Health risks are similar, so please make sure to consult your doctor before beginning any yoga practice, especially one in an intensely heated environment.

SIX - Letting Go

None of the medications and dietary changes I tried seemed to help me; I could no longer ignore the idea that stress might be what was causing my acid reflux. As I mentioned earlier, I never thought of myself as stressed. It took a while to realize that my emotions were the main reason for my health problems. Stress was the term used, but I did not feel like I was stressed. What they should have said was emotional, or unhappy. Emotions such as depression, anger and resentment can have serious health consequences.

The first thing my yoga teacher taught me was to **let go**. I simply needed to stop getting upset. Unhappy thoughts can make us very sick.

This might be difficult at first, but you have to find a way to let things go if you want to be healthy and happy in this life. If you see something upsetting, do not dwell on it. Try to focus on a thought, any thought that stirs up even a slightly more positive emotion. Trust me, I get it. I live and drive in Los Angeles. Road rage comes delivered with the morning coffee in LA. Not all of us can flip the switch from <u>rage</u> to <u>love</u> on command. It would be ridiculous to expect anyone to do that without practice. If you could just take the leap from "You idiot!" to "I like that song that just started playing on the radio," it might make a big difference in your life. If that seems too far to stretch, you could try switching from rage to anger. That is a tad easier, is it not? The point is, as long as you are moving in the direction of positive emotions, you are on the right track. Shortening the amount of time it takes to get there requires practice.

Once you have managed to escape that rush of negative emotions (be it seconds, minutes, days or years), you can take a step back from the situation. Try to see everything from a distance, both visually and emotionally, like a hawk floating in the sky, witnessing events unfold below you. See the event through the eyes of an uninterested third party, having no feeling, no weight and no worries about how anything below you turns out. Witness yourself; participate in the action that unfolds below. That is the only secret to being happy that really exists. As long as you are trying, you are winning. If you struggle to detach yourself from a negative event, consider this: You are hanging on to something that is poisoning you. The person who suffers the consequences of your negative emotion is you, nobody else. If you look at it like that, it might finally seem not worth holding on to.

Whenever there is an argument forming with a friend, family member or co-worker, I do not dig my heels in and get ready to protect my point of view. I usually walk away, take a few minutes and, when I am calm, I come back to fix the problem. I could not always do that before. It was only through repeated practice and making positive choices in thought, one step after another, that I finally reached that state.

Do you know a person who always has to be right and have the last word, who argues over everything, with everyone? I have met people like this. They were generally unhappy, in a bad mood and irritable. No one wanted to spend time in their presence. Did this person, in your opinion, have good health, or do you think they were bothered by aches and pains? If you asked, would they say that all the problems, the aches and pains, came before the bad mood? Do you think that is true? Maybe you have a tendency to be like this, as I once did.

SEVEN - Pranayama & Asana

Pranayama is one of the eight limbs (or branches) of yoga, as defined in The Yoga Sutras of Patanjali, one of the primary texts of Ashtanga Yoga (also known as raja yoga). The word pranayama comes from the Sanskrit words prana (breath) and ayama (to extend or draw out), and literally means extension of breath.

According to B.K.S. Iyengar, one of the world's leading yoga teachers, pranayama is a conscious prolongation of inhalation and exhalation. The Bhagavad Gita describes pranayama as a "trance to end all breathing." It is, in other words, an exercise designed to progressively lengthen and extend your breath, sometimes to the point where it seems there is no breath at all.

Pranayama breathing exercises can increase the volume of air brought into the lungs, allowing more oxygen to enter your body.

In general, most people breathe very shallow, lazy, thoughtless breaths. Pranayama is the exact opposite—it is breathing full, focused, intentional breaths.

What is prana, and why do we need it? One might assume the benefits of pranayama to be limited to the physical intake of more air into the lungs, and the benefits of extra oxygen. However, from a yogic perspective, prana is much more than just the air we breathe in and out of us. Prana, according to Yogi Bhajan (the introducer of kundalini yoga to the United States), "is the most powerful and creative thing God ever created, because out of prana came life." Prana is energy, the energy that all life comes from. Personally, I like to call it energy or life force. When I do my breathing exercises, I am using this energy to nourish and heal my body.

It is best to do pranayama or any yoga practice on an empty stomach, or at least an hour after eating. It is better to have a regular schedule of practice, even if it is a short session once every day, as opposed to taking a class once a week. I like to start my day with a pranayama practice. Sometimes I do another session later in the day before lunch.

Prana is in every living thing. It is the source of life. Without prana, there is no life. Prana is in the air, but it is not air. It is in food and water, but it is not food or water. The air is full of prana, which people can absorb by normal breathing. By deep breathing, and even more so by yogic breathing, you can get so much prana that you will have enough to store for later. This concept may sound silly, but it reminds me of the fat-soluble vitamins, like vitamin D. These vitamins are stored in the body, unlike water-soluble vitamins like vitamin C, which empty out if you get more than you can use immediately. When walking on a nice sunny day, I think about how I am replenishing my storages of the sunshine vitamin. Similarly, when you practice yogic breathing you can fill the stores of prana, this positive, healing energy. It is very important, however, that you start slowly and do not overdo it. Too much, too soon, can cause more harm than good.

Few people know how to breathe correctly; we only use a small portion of our lung capacity. I am no exception. Until I learned about yogic breathing, I had no idea how much air I could inhale into my lungs—how big and extensive they are. Most women only breathe at the top of the chest, and most men only practice low abdominal breathing. This is barely enough to survive; nobody can thrive on that. Think about how important it is to breathe. You can live without food for several weeks, months in some cases, and without water for a few days, but how long can you go without air? A minute or two, maybe? You will not understand what a huge difference these exercises make until you experience it yourself. Breathing alone can restore health in a person. Yoga says that true healing can never come about from an outside source, only by waking up the healing force inside.

According to yoga wisdom, the only way to get an immune system strong enough to keep us from getting sick and allow us to live long is by mastering our breathing. Lazy breathing will give us a shorter life, low energy/vitality and less happiness, and make us catch even the mildest colds that come our way.

Among other things, a regular practice of pranayama can help regulate your weight, whether you are under or overweight. It will help manage stress and related illnesses (blood pressure, heart conditions, overeating), can help relieve asthma symptoms, reduces the signs of oxidative stress in the body, can extend life and enhance the quality of life, and improves mood and one's general outlook.

Swimming as Breathing Exercise

If you find that pranayama is too hard or complicated, try swimming instead, or in addition to the practice. It is a natural way of exercising, and it can have the same benefits as a regular pranayama practice. As long as you swim with your head in the water, not the trying to preserve my hair-do kind of way. Be mindful while swimming. Exhale fully at the start to make room for the fresh air, then inhale deep, hold it when you go under water, exhale fully under water, and when the head comes above water take another deep inhale. The breaststroke works best, swimming very slowly, like a meditation. Swimming can gently strengthen the muscles, and it may benefit spinal issues. It will also have all the same benefits of pranayama: regulate weight, helps digestive issues and increases mood and physical well-being.

Breathing Exercises

The first practice we look at is the Complete Breath. You can do this standing or sitting, but may find it easier lying down. The benefits include waking and warming the body, reducing anxiety and improving focus and concentration. On a cold morning, I sometimes practice it before getting out of bed, as it helps me warm up.

Complete Yoga Breathing Warm-Ups

The first part is the lower breath. Always breathe through the nose during this practice, since prana is not absorbed through the mouth.

Step 1: Place the hands on the chest or belly.

Step 2: Take seven slow deep breaths. Expand the belly on every inhale and pull it back in on every exhale. Push all the old air out to make room for new air and new prana to heal and nourish.

The second part is the middle breath.

Step 1: Move one hand to the upper belly and the other up to the collarbone.

Step 2: Breathe seven times in and out, slowly and deeply feeling the lower ribs expanding.

The third is the upper breath

Step 1: Move the hands down and rest them the lower belly.

Step 2: Breathe into the top part of the chest, seven times. After the warm-ups are done, move on to the Complete Yoga Breath.

Complete Yoga Breath

Step 1: Place the hands on the heart, and feel it beating.

Step 2: Empty the lungs completely. Slowly breathe in, starting at the lower belly and filling up toward the collarbone.

Step 3: Count eight heartbeats for the inhale and eight for the exhale. If this is difficult, try four heartbeats and gradually increase.
Step 4: Repeat seven times.

Complete Yoga Breath with Hold

Step 1: Place hands on heart.

Step 2: Breathe in for a count of eight. Again, if this is difficult, start with a count of four and gradually increase.

Step 3: Hold the air in for as long as possible.

Step 4: When you are ready to exhale, let the air out slowly through the nostrils while counting to eight.

Step 5: Repeat three times only, no matter how much you want to do more. Keep in mind that doing too much too soon might cause more harm than good.

Yoga Poses

Ardha Matsyendrasana - Half Lord of the Fishes (Spinal Twist)

Pose benefits: Improves digestion and elimination of wastes, stretches, massages and rejuvenates the spine, strengthens the abdominals and oblique, and massages and stimulates the internal organs. It can even correct scoliosis.

Contraindications: If you have any recent or chronic hip, shoulder or back injuries, only practice this pose under the supervision of an experienced teacher.

Version One

Step 1: Sit on a folded blanket or towel to support the lower back, legs extended.

Step 2: Sitting tall, bend the left knee, placing the left foot on the floor next to the right knee.

Step 3: Place the right hand on the floor behind you, fingers pointing away.

Step 4: Bring the left elbow to the inside of the left knee and the fingertips to the right knee, gently pressing the left knee to the left elbow and the fingertips to the right knee.

Step 5: Inhale, lengthening the spine upwards.
Step 6: Exhale, pulling the abdominals in to the spine and gently turning towards the right to look over the right shoulder.

Step 7: Keep the hips stable, turning from the middle spine.

Step 8: Hold for 30 seconds or however long is comfortable, then release on an exhale.

Step 9: Repeat on the second side.

Version Two

Step 1: Sit on the floor with your legs extended.

Step 2: Bend the left leg at the knee and set the heel firmly against the perineum.

Step 3: Bend the right leg at the knee. Lifting it from the floor with the support of the hands, place the right foot to the outside of the left thigh, so that the right outer ankle touches the left thigh. Spend a little time in this position, keeping the shin perpendicular to the floor.

Step 4: Turn the torso 90 degrees to the right on an exhale, so that the left armpit touches the outer side of the knee.

Step 5: Reach the left hand around the right knee to firmly catch the right big toe with the left hand.

Step 6: Swing the right hand around the back to the left side of the waist to catch the left thigh.

Step 7: Turn the head to the right shoulder, directing the gaze over it.

Step 8: Remain in this posture, maintaining normal breathing, for 30 seconds, working up to a few minutes

Step 9: Repeat this process on the other side.

Uddiyana Bandha - Upward Lock (Belly Squeeze)

The following are three variations of the same idea. Feel free to choose the one you are most comfortable with, or you may do all three. We will be contracting our abdominal muscles.

Version One

Step 1: Sit cross-legged, or in lotus.

Step 2: Bring the hands behind the back, clasping the left wrist with the right hand.

Step 3: Inhale. On the exhale, bend forward, placing the forehead on the floor in front of the knees.

Step 4: Push all the air out of the lungs; squeeze the abdominal muscles, pulling them in and up.

Step 5: Hold for as long as comfortable.

Step 6: Inhale to come up, returning to the beginning position.

Step 7: Follow this with one cycle (in and out) of normal breathing.

Step 8: Repeat three times.

Version Two

Step 1: Sit on the heels. Placing the hands on the knees or thighs, wherever feels comfortable.

Step 2: Inhale, then exhale fully, squeezing the abdominal muscles and pulling them up and in.

Step 3: Hold for a few seconds.

Step 4: Release the muscles to inhale again.

Step 5: Follow with one cycle of normal breathing and repeat two more times.

Version Three

The third variation is from Tim Ferris' book The Four Hour Body. His focus is building six-pack abdominals. He calls it the heaving cat or the cat vomit. In yoga, it is usually goes by the name of the cat/cow sequence.

Step 1: Come to your hands and knees.

Step 2: Inhale. As you exhale, squeeze the muscles in the abdomen.

Step 3: Hold for a few seconds, then inhale as you release.

Step 4: Follow with a full cycle of breath in between repetitions.

When I tried his version, it felt good, so I added it to my regular practice. You can pick your favorite, do all three or switch it up based on your mood that day.

Nadi Shodhana - Channel Clearing (Alternate Nostril Breathing)

Nadi shodhana clears our blocked energy channels in the body, which in turn calms the mind. It also improves brain function. It is a good tool to use before an exam or interview.

Step 1: Begin sitting cross-legged or in any comfortable position.

Step 2: Touch the thumb and forefinger of the left hand together. Place the hand down comfortably, with the back of the hand on the left knee.

Step 3: Place the right forefinger on the forehead.

Step 4: Hold the right nostril closed with the right thumb.

Step 5: Inhale through the left nostril for a count of four.

Step 6: Hold the breath for 4, 8 or 16 counts (it gets easier with more practice).

Step 7: Place the ring finger on the left nostril and exhale through the right for the same count.

Step 8: Inhale through the right nostril, then hold the air in.

Step 9: When ready to exhale, switch the finger and let the air out through the left nostril on an eight count.

Step 10: Repeat three times.

There you have it. It's that simple! Anybody can learn to do this, and it only takes seven minutes.

EIGHT - Meditation

Meditation, known as dharana (concentration) and dhyana (meditation) by yoga practitioners, is a great way to release stress and improve your mood in general. These are two of the eight limbs of yoga described by Patanjali, but by no means does meditation need to be a spiritual practice. The East as well as the West has extensively studied its benefits. The long list of reasons to do it includes reducing stress, decreasing anxiety, slowing the aging process, improving the immune system and increasing happiness. I do it because it feels good and makes me happier.

Initially, meditation was difficult. I had a hard time focusing and my mind kept wandering. I tried many different types and methods of meditation, and the one thing I found most useful was listening to guided meditations and/or binaural beats. Wearing headphones keeps most people from sitting down and starting to chat with you, and the guided audio helps keep the mind from racing. I needed something to focus on other than my breathing. If you are not familiar with binaural beats, they may help induce meditative and relaxation stages by synchronizing the brain wave cycles to lower frequencies associated with these stages. Scientists are still working on finding conclusive evidence of the benefits, but I find it to be extremely helpful.

Conclusion

I could have written a long book about all the medications and commonly used home remedies for heartburn. I could have told you about the beneficial effects of honey and apple cider vinegar, baking soda, milk and apples. But I did not see any value in doing that. There are countless books and Web pages out there where you can learn that information. If any of those remedies work for you, that is great. However, it is still only a temporary solution. By practicing a few breathing exercises for only seven minutes every day you could be heartburn free for the rest of your life. Isn't that an amazing thought?

I hope you enjoyed reading this book as much I enjoyed writing it. It is something I have wanted to do for a long time. When I finally found the answer to my struggle with heartburn, my life changed for the better, and I feel that I have to share this answer with fellow sufferers out there. Remember, this simple seven-minute solution can change your life too.

About the Author

I want to tell you a little bit more about me. Obviously, I am a big fan of yoga, but I also enjoy traveling, swimming, Pilates, Krav-Maga, Zumba, backpacking and running (although my endurance is not where I'd like it to be). Oddly, I really do not enjoy cycling at all—but maybe someday! Oh, and yes, I used to be a professional ballerina.

I love to read about health and nutrition. I do not watch, read or listen to the news. I find it too depressing, so I only watch funny, uplifting movies. I generally try to find things that make me happy. I truly think that you can find a way to be happy in every moment of every day. It just takes a little practice.

My newest challenge is to find a way to never say anything negative about anybody or anything. I am still working on this one.

I almost forgot, I love cats.

A Message from the Author

Dear Reader,

Thank you very much for purchasing this book. We hope you enjoyed reading this book as much as we did writing it.

There are many more books to come in this great series, and we hope you continue to read along as we continue to explore the world of natural and alternative healing.

 If you learned something new, or benefited from reading this book in some way, we ask that you take a few seconds and leave us a review. Reviews help our books reach a wider audience and encourage us to keep adding more books to this series.

Thank you again.

Wishing you the best,
Mae

Bibliography

Cowan, D. (n.d.). Emotions and the Endocrine Glands, Natural Alternatives for Health & Wellness.

Ferriss, T. (2010). The Four-Hour Body. New York: Random House.

Fuerstein, G. (n.d.). A Short History of Yoga. Traditional Yoga and Meditation of the Himalayan Masters.

Haich, S. Y. (1953). Sport es Yoga. Lazi Konyvkiado Kft.

Iyengar, B. (1966). Light on Yoga. New York: Schocken Books.

M.D., T. M. (2007). Yoga as Medicine. New York: Bantam Dell.

PhD, S. F. (1999). Nourishing Traditions; The Cookbook that Changes Politically Correct Nutrition and the Diet Dictocrats. Washington DC: New Trends Publishing.

Sedlock vs. Timothy Baird Superintendent. CASE NO: 37-2013-00035910-CU-MC-CTL. (2013, July 1). Superior Court of California.

Semmelweis Society International. (n.d.). Dr. Semmelweis Biography. Semmelweis Society International, semmelweis.org.